Low Carb Cookbook

Delicious & Simple Low Carb High Fat Ketogenic Recipes Meal Plan

(High Protein Low Carb Recipes)

Published by Jason Thawne Publishing House

© Conrad Spencer

Low Carb Cookbook: Delicious & Simple Low Carb High Fat Ketogenic Recipes Meal Plan

(High Protein Low Carb Recipes)

All Rights Reserved

ISBN 978-1-989749-34-0

This document is geared towards providing exact and reliable information in regards to the topic and issue covered. The publication is sold with the idea that the publisher isn't required to render accounting, officially permitted, or otherwise, qualified services. If advice is necessary, legal or even professional, a practiced individual in the profession should be ordered.

- From a Declaration of Principles which was accepted and approved equally by a Committee of the American Bar Association and a Committee of Publishers and Associations.

In no way is it legal to reproduce, duplicate, or even transmit any part of this document in either electronic means or in printed format. Recording of this publication is strictly prohibited and any storage of this document isn't allowed unless with proper written permission from the publisher. All rights reserved.

The information provided herein is stated to be truthful and consistent, in that any liability, in terms of inattention or otherwise, by any usage or abuse of any policies, processes, or directions contained within is the solitary and also utter responsibility of the recipient reader. Under no circumstances will any legal responsibility or blame be held against the publisher for any reparation, damages, or monetary loss due to the information herein, either directly or indirectly.

Respective authors own all copyrights not held by the publisher.

The information herein is offered for just informational purposes solely, and is universal as so. The presentation of the information is without contract or any type of guarantee assurance.

The trademarks that are used are without any consent, and also the publication of the trademark is without permission or backing by the trademark owner. All trademarks and brands within this book are for clarifying purposes only and are the owned by the owners themselves, not affiliated with this document.

TABLE OF CONTENTS

Part 1 1

Low Carb Breakfasts 1

Artichoke Shrimp Frittata 1

Cream Cheese And Omelet 3

Chicken Sausage Sweet Potato Hash 5

Swiss Chard And Ricotta Pie 6

Low Carb Main Dishes 8

Baked Meatball Sensation 8

Beef Stroganoff 10

Ancho Macho Chili Delight 12

Gravy And Turkey Delight 14

Chili And Orange Chicken Delight 17

Low Carb Desserts 19

Tasty Brownies 19

Sugar-Free Chocolate Peanut Butter Fudge 20

Lemon Cheesecake 21

Raspberry Jell O 24

Low Carb Snacks 26

Shrimp And Cucumber Rounds 26

Eggplant Chips 27

Cayenne Deviled Eggs 29

Parmesan Chips 30

Conclusion 32

Part 2 33

Introduction 34

Chapter 1 - Why Low Carb Mediterranean Dieting? 36

Chapter 2 - What To Eat And What To Avoid 43

Chapter 3 - Sides And Dressings 45

Vinaigrette 45

Kale Side Dish 46

Low-Carb Tzatziki Sauce 47

Chapter 4 - Salads And Lighter Fare 50

Turkey Tomato Bowl 51

Blt Wraps 53

Chicken Fajita Lettuce Wraps 54

Light Salad 56

Stuffed Tomatoes 57

Garbanzo Bean Salad 58

Tuna Salad 59

Quinoa Salad 60

Simple Caprese Salad 62

Halibut Salad 62

Chapter 5 - Heartier Meals 65

Mediterranean Chicken 65

Steak And Olives 66

Basic Breakfast 67

Shish-Kabob Skewers 68

Chickpea Patties 69

Simple And Delicious Salmon 71

Stuffed Mushrooms 72

Roasted Red Pepper 74

Rosemary Chicken 76

Chapter 6 - Weekly Meal Plan And Daily Shopping Lists 79

Conclusion 87

About The Author 88

PART 1

LOW CARB BREAKFASTS

ARTICHOKE SHRIMP FRITTATA

Ingredients

½ (9-ounce) package frozen artichoke hearts

4 ounces fresh shrimp in shells

¼ cup fat-free milk

12 eggs, beaten

3 tablespoons parmesan cheese, finely shredded

1/8 teaspoon garlic powder

¼ cup green onions, thinly sliced

Non-stick cooking spray

1/8 teaspoon pepper

Optional

Cherry tomatoes, quartered

Parsley.

Instructions

Devein the shrimp, rinse and pat dry. Half the shrimp lengthwise, season with salt and pepper then put aside. In the mean time, cook the artichoke hearts depending on the package directions then drain, and cut them into quarters and put aside.

Stir together the milk, eggs, garlic powder, onions and pepper then put aside.

Coat a non-stick pan with cooking spray then heat until a drop of water sizzles. Add shrimp to pan and cook for one to three minutes until the shrimp is opaque.

Pour the egg mixture into the skillet on low heat and do not stir the eggs. As the egg sets, run a spatula on the edge of the skillet and lift the edge to let the liquid run underneath. Cook until the mixture is almost set.

Remove from heat, sprinkle with artichoke hearts and Parmesan cheese on the top and allow this to stand for four minutes then transfer to a serving plate. Garnish with the parsley and cherry tomatoes.

Nutritional Information

Servings: 4

Calories: 126

Carbs: 6g

CREAM CHEESE AND OMELET

Ingredients

4 eggs

1 tablespoon olive oil

2 tablespoons water

2 tablespoons minced chives

2 ounces cream cheese, cubed

1/8 teaspoon pepper

1/8 teaspoon salt

Salsa

Instructions

Heat oil in a large pan over medium heat. Whisk eggs, water, chives, pepper and salt. Add this mixture to the skillet.

As eggs set, push them towards the center to ensure that the uncooked portion goes beneath. Immediately the eggs set, sprinkle cream cheese on one side then fold egg over the filling. Slide this onto a plate cut into half and serve with salsa.

Nutritional Information Per Serving

Servings: 2

Calories (without salsa): 305

Carbs (without salsa): 2g

CHICKEN SAUSAGE SWEET POTATO HASH

Ingredients

1 sweet potato, diced

3 ounces red bell pepper, diced

3 ounces yellow bell pepper, diced

5 ounces onion, diced

1 lb chicken sausage

1 large green onion, chopped

4 tablespoons olive oil, divided

Salt and pepper

2 cloves garlic, minced

Instructions

Heat two tablespoons of olive oil in a pan over medium heat. Once pan is hot, add the diced sweet potatoes, garlic and pepper then cook until the sweet potatoes are tender and nicely browned. As the sweet potatoes are cooking, heat another two tablespoons of olive oil in a skillet on medium heat. Once oil is heated, add the onions, chicken sausage pepper and salt and cook until the onions are no longer pink and the sausage is translucent and soft.

Combine ingredients from both pans, garnish with green onions then serve.

Nutritional Information Per serving

Serving: 1

Calories: 214

Carbs: 8 net g

Swiss Chard and Ricotta Pie

Ingredients

½ cup onion, chopped

1 tablespoon olive oil

8 cups Swiss chard, chopped

1 clove garlic, minced

1 lb sausage

1/8 teaspoon ground nutmeg

¼ cup Parmesan cheese, shredded

Salt and pepper to taste

3 eggs

2 cups whole milk ricotta cheese

1 cup mozzarella cheese, shredded

Instructions

Preheat oven to 350 degrees F then heat olive oil in a large pan then add garlic and onion and cook until soft. Add the Swiss chard and cook for five minutes until the leaves are wilted. Add nutmeg and season with salt and pepper. Remove from heat and set aside to cool.

In the mean time, beat eggs in a bowl, add the ricotta, mozzarella and parmesan cheeses and stir. Roll out the sausage and press it into a pie tin then pour the filling and place on a cookie sheet to catch any dripping of oil from the sausage. Bake for 30-35 minutes or until firm.

Nutritional Information per serving

Serving: 8

Calories: 230

Carbs: 1.3 net g

Low Carb Main Dishes

Baked Meatball Sensation

Ingredients

½ finely chopped green onion

3 cloves of minced garlic

2 eggs

½ teaspoon of salt

¼ teaspoon of pepper

½ cup of grated parmesan cheese

1 tablespoon of olive oil

½ pound of ground veal

½ pound of ground pork

½ pound of ground beef

Instructions

Preheat the oven to 375 ° F. Cook the onions over high heat in a skillet for five minutes while stirring frequently. Then stir in the garlic and cook for one more minute. Transfer the onion and garlic to a bowl and mix in the ground meat, salt, pepper and eggs. Next, roll mixture into ball-sized meatballs and place them on a jelly roll pan. Finally bake them for twenty to twenty five minutes until they are brown and thoroughly cooked.

Nutritional Information Per Serving

Serves: 4

Carbs: 2g

Calories: 409

BEEF STROGANOFF

Ingredients

2 tablespoons of canola oil

1/8 teaspoon of pepper

1/8 teaspoon of salt

1 ¼ pounds of beef tenderloin, cut into strips

½ cup of finely chopped Spanish onion

1 tablespoon of butter

¼ cup of sour cream

¼ cup of dry wine

3 ounces of small, white mushrooms

1 cup of beef broth

1 teaspoon of Dijon mustard

Instructions

Heat oven to warm setting and sprinkle the meat with pepper and salt. Heat the oil over a medium-high heat in a large, non-stick skillet. Brown the meat in batches for about one minute per side and then transfer them to a platter and place them in the oven then melt the butter in a skillet and then onions and cook them for three minutes. Later add the mushrooms and cook them for ten minutes while constantly stirring until the mushroom liquid has evaporated. Add the wine to the mix and cook for five minutes and then put in the beef broth and cook for about ten minutes until the mushrooms are completely coated in sauce. At this point, you may stir in the mustard and sour cream and then add the meat and accumulated juices. Finally reduce the heat to a low setting and cook for two to three minutes until all the meat is heated through. At this point, you may also add your salt and pepper to taste.

Nutritional Information Per Serving

Serves: 4

Calories: 379

Carbs: 3.5g

A**NCHO** M**ACHO** C**HILI DELIGHT**

Ingredients

2 teaspoons of kosher salt

4 large roasted and minced garlic cloves

¾ cup of chicken broth or dry red wine

1 chopped medium yellow onion

½ teaspoon of freshly grounded black pepper

3 tablespoons of Mexican styled chili powder

3 tablespoons of canola oil, divided

1 (14 ½ ounce) can of tomatoes diced and mixed with green chiles

5 pounds of beef chuck stew meet which has been deboned and cut into 1 ½ inch cubes

Instructions

Heat the oven to 325 °F. Toss the beef with pepper and salt and one and a half teaspoons of the oil in a Dutch oven over high heat. Add about a third of the beef and brown it on all sides for about five minutes. Then transfer this to a bowl and repeat the process two or more times with the beef and the oil. Cook the onion in the last 1 ½ teaspoons of oil in the Dutch oven and then stir in the tomatoes, wine, garlic and chile powder and bring it to a simmer. Next, return the beef with its accumulated juices to the oven. Cover it and cook for the next two and a half hours until the beef is tender. Finally, garnish with shredded cheese, green onions or sour cream.

Nutritional Information Per Serving

Serves: 10

Calories: 325

Carbs: 3.5g

GRAVY AND TURKEY DELIGHT

Ingredients

1 cup of chicken broth

1 tablespoon of thick-it-up

½ celery stalk, halved

1 tablespoon of poultry seasoning

2 smashed garlic cloves

2 to 3 parsley sprigs

Black pepper corns

Bay leaf

1 cup of water

12 pounds of whole turkey (with the giblets reserved) rinsed, defrosted and patted dry

Instructions

Heat the oven to 325°C. Put the turkey on a rack in a large shallow roasting pan then season the turkey with poultry seasoning, salt and pepper then add water to the pan. Then roast the turkey, basting it occasionally with the pan drippings and you should add more water if the pan gets dry. Continue doing this until an instant-read thermometer when inserted into the thigh (but not touching the thighbone) measures 175°F to 180°F. The stuffing should also register 165°F. You may cover the turkey loosely with a heavy duty foil during the last hour of cooking to prevent it from getting too brown. When you have finished doing that, remove the turkey and put it on a cutting board. Let it cool for twenty to thirty minutes before you carve it.

To make the gravy, combine the water, giblets, garlic, parsley, celery, peppercorn and bay leaf in a large saucepan and bring it to boil over high heat, while ensuring you skim off the foam that rises to the surface. Turn down the heat and let it simmer until it is reduced to about 2 cups. You may dice the giblets if you like and remove the meat from the neck of the turkey to so that it can be added to the gravy. Then strain and wrap in plastic, refrigerate the broth and giblets until you are ready to use them.

Pour the juices obtained from the roasting pan into a glass measure and skim off the fat. Then add the giblet broth to measure three cups. Add the chicken broth, if it is needed. Place the roasting pan over two burners on the stovetop. Add the pan-juice mixture and bring it to a boil over medium heat. Then stir in the thick-it-up thickener, giblets and neck meat whilst ensuring that you stir regularly. Reduce the heat to a low setting and let it simmer for about five minutes. Season with the pepper and salt to your preference and carve the turkey and serve with the stuffing and gravy.

Nutritional Information Per Serving

Serves: 16

Calories: 426.5

Carbs: 0.6g

CHILI AND ORANGE CHICKEN DELIGHT

Ingredients

1 teaspoon of granular sugar substitute, such as sucralose

1 tablespoon of extra virgin olive oil

¼ cup of fresh olive oil

2 teaspoons of chopped garlic

1 tablespoon of chili powder

1 teaspoon of grated orange peel

¼ teaspoon of cayenne pepper

2 pounds of chicken breasts

Instructions

Mix the orange juice, garlic, oil, sugar substitute, chili powder, cayenne pepper and orange rind in a large, re-sealable plastic bag. Add the chicken breasts and toss it to coat them. Refrigerate this mixture overnight.

The next day, heat the broiler and season the chicken with pepper and salt. Position the broiler rack so that it is six inches from the heat source and broil the chicken for twelve to fifteen minutes, turning it half way through the cooking time until it is cooked through.

Nutritional Information Per Serving

Serves: 4

Calories: 430.5

Carbs: 2.2g

Low Carb Desserts

Tasty Brownies

Ingredients

2 cups powdered erythritol

¼ lb butter

4 eggs

1 tablespoon vanilla

1 teaspoon salt

½ cup cocoa

2/3 cup water

1/3 cup cream

1 tablespoon baking powder

2 cups flaxseed meal

4 ounces unsweetened chocolate, melted

1 cup walnuts (optional)

Instructions

Beat the butter until fluffy then add the erythritol to the butter and beat until well combined.

Add vanilla and eggs one at a time while beating. Then add cocoa, salt and chocolate and beat until fluffy.

Add the other ingredients and mix well to combine. Pour the mixture into a pan and bake for 35-40 minutes.

Allow this to cool then cut into 32 squares.

Nutritional Information Per Brownie

Yield: 32 Brownies

Calories: 107

Carbs: 1g

Sugar-Free Chocolate Peanut Butter Fudge

Ingredients

8 ounces unsweetened chocolate

¾ cup erythritol

½ teaspoon vanilla

1 cup peanut butter (without sugar)

Pinch of salt

1 cup liquid sucralose

Instructions

Melt chocolate then add in the other ingredients. Spread on a loaf pan and put in the refrigerator. Once set cut into 18 pieces and serve.

Nutritional Information Per Piece

Yield: 18 Pieces

Calories: 146

Carbs: 3g

LEMON CHEESECAKE

Ingredients

Crust

2 tablespoons melted butter

1 ¼ cups almond meal

3 tablespoons of artificial sweetener

Filling

1 ¼ cups splenda

1 ½ lbs cream cheese at room temperature

¼ teaspoon salt

1 ½ teaspoons vanilla extract

4 eggs

¼ cup heavy cream

1 tablespoon lemon zest

¼ cup lemon juice

Topping

½ teaspoon vanilla extract

1 cup sour cream

Juice and zest of a medium lemon

¼ cup artificial sweetener

Instructions

Preheat the oven to 375º F. Put parchment paper at the bottom of the pan then butter the sides and bottom of the pan.

Mix the crust ingredients and press this mixture into the pan and bake for 10 minutes then remove from oven.

Beat the cream cheese until fluffy then add vanilla, salt, sweetener and two of the eggs then beat and scrape down the mixture then add the other two eggs and beat well.

Add lemon zest, cream and lemon juice and beat well then pour this filling into the pan over the crust.

In another bowl, mix the ingredients for the topping and put aside. Place a baking pan that is large enough to hold your pie pan and fill it halfway with boiling water then place pan into the larger baking pan and bake for 10 to 15 minutes until the cheesecake is almost set.

Remove from oven, spread toping and bake for an additional ten minutes. Allow this to cool to room temperature or chill for several minutes before you serve.

Nutritional Information per Piece

Serving: 16

Calories: 295

Carbs: 3g

RASPBERRY JELL O

Ingredients

1 cup cold water

2 cups apple-raspberry juice

2 cups raspberries, divided

1 cup apple juice

1/3 cup sugar

4 envelopes unflavored gelatin

Instructions

Bring raspberry juice to a boil in a pan over high heat. In the mean time, pour water in a large heatproof bowl then sprinkle gelatin over the water and then let this stand for about 3 minutes. Add the juice and stir to ensure that the gelatin is completely dissolved. Add the sugar and stir until dissolved.

Whisk in the apple juice. Refrigerate the mixture until you achieve a thin pudding like consistency and is just starting to set around the edges. After an hour of refrigeration, start checking every 10 minutes since it thickens quickly after that.

When thick, whisk this mixture gently but thoroughly until uniform then stir in the raspberries and pour this into a pan, cover with plastic wrap and refrigerate for three hours. If your finger does not stick to the jell-o then it is done.

Run a small knife round the edge of the pan and cut into 16 squares

Nutritional Information Per square

Serving: 16

Calories: 53

Carbs: 12g

LOW CARB SNACKS

SHRIMP AND CUCUMBER ROUNDS

Ingredients

½ lb cooked shrimp, peeled, deveined and chopped finely

2 green onions, sliced thinly

½ cup reduced-fat mayonnaise

Dash of cayenne pepper

1 teaspoon dill pickle relish

1 celery stalk, finely chopped

1 cucumber cut into a quarter inch slices

Instructions

Combine the first six ingredients in a small bowl and spoon onto cucumber slices.

Nutritional Information Per Appetizer

Yield: 36

Calories: 20

Carbs: 1g

EGGPLANT CHIPS

Ingredients

¼ cup grated Parmesan Cheese

1 eggplant, unpeeled and thinly sliced into rounds

1 tablespoon garlic powder

1 teaspoon leaves Italian seasoning

1 tablespoon olive oil

Instructions

Preheat oven to 375ºF. Pour the olive oil on cookie sheet and sprinkle with garlic powder. Swoosh the cookie sheet in order to mix and coat sheet well.

Place the eggplant slices on the cookie sheet. Rub each slice into the garlic powder and olive oil coated cookie sheet and turn each slice over and rub the other side.

Sprinkle lightly with the parmesan cheese and Italian seasoning and turn over gently to sprinkle parmesan cheese and Italian seasoning on the other side.

Bake these for around 10-15 minutes. Ensure that you watch the eggplant slices closely until they are nicely browned on each side. The time may be longer depending on the thickness of the eggplant slices

Nutritional Information Per serving

Serving: 3

Calories: 123

Carbs: 11.58

CAYENNE DEVILED EGGS

Ingredients

3 tablespoons mayonnaise

2 teaspoons Dijon mustard

2 teaspoons cayenne

1 teaspoon mustard seed

1 teaspoon chili powder

8 hard boiled eggs

Instructions

Cut eggs in half and remove yolks then put in a bowl and mush up to avoid big lumps in the filling.

Add mustard and mayonnaise slowly to the egg yolks and mix as you go. Add the cayenne and chilli to the mixture as you taste then add the mustard seed ensuring that you mix thoroughly.

Take the yolk mixture and fill the eggs, sprinkle some cayenne on top and serve.

Nutritional Information Per Serving

Serves: 16

Calories: 62

Carbs: 0.57g

Parmesan Chips

Ingredients

½ cup Parmesan cheese, grated

Instructions

Heat an 8-inch pan over medium heat then sprinkle half the cheese in the pan evenly forming some sort of pancake.

Leave the "pancake" for two minutes until melted then flip using a spatula. Brown the other side and remove from pan to a cutting board. While still warm, cut into triangles using a sharp knife. Do the same for the remaining cheese.

Nutritional Information Per serving

Serves: 2

Calories: 108

Carbohydrates: 1.02g

Conclusion

Thank you again for downloading this book!

I hope this book has helped you to know how you can lose weight with the low carb diet

The next step is to start trying the recipes outlined in this book and watch those pounds drop off.

Part 2

Introduction

This book contains proven steps and strategies on how to follow a low-carb Mediterranean-style diet while eating delicious and simple foods that will make you feel great.

In this book, you will find plenty of information to help you understand why low-carb dieting works, and why the Mediterranean diet specifically can adapt so well to a low-carb lifestyle. You will be able to choose healthy food options from a list of food categories you should consume, while learning all about the types of foods you should avoid eating. The last few chapters of the book also provide you with twenty-five tasty recipes to keep on hand for your lunches, dinners, and side dishes, as well as a week-long meal plan that should help you transition to your new diet.

Thanks again for downloading this book, I hope you enjoy it!

Chapter 1 - Why Low Carb Mediterranean Dieting?

Low-carb dieting has been around for a long time now. The Atkins diet started the fad, but ever since then, many other diets have caught on to the fact that carbohydrates are not necessary, and in fact cause significant weight gain when eaten in large quantities.

Low-carb dieting follows the concept that reducing the consumption and daily intake of carbohydrates will help lower the daily production of insulin. This causes the body to deplete fat stores in order to compensate, which leads to quick and effective weight loss.

Basically, the body uses carbohydrates first as an energy source. When carbohydrates are restricted, it is forced to go to the next available option, which is proteins. A low-carb diet relies heavily on increased amounts of protein to help balance the body's metabolism and provide plenty of energy when carbs are unavailable. After the protein has been burned, the body must then turn to the last available source of energy: fat. This is when the fat will start to melt away as the body burns it for necessary energy.

This process is known as ketosis, and when induced with a balanced diet to offset the lack of carbs, it is a healthy and beneficial way to lose weight fast.

Low-carb dieting also focuses on foods that are sure to help you fill up fast and keep that full feeling for longer than foods that are high in carbs. Carbohydrate-heavy foods are burned off quickly, and so they do not make you feel full and energetic for as long as do protein-rich foods. You will not have as much of an appetite while eating low-carb foods, which will help you lose weight even faster.

Mediterranean style recipes fit snugly into the concept of low-carb dieting simply by their very nature. Mediterranean food makes excellent use of olive oil, which is a very healthy, natural form of oil low in carbs and high in nutritional value. Most Mediterranean dishes already revolve around a basic protein, such as beef or chicken, and therefore are very useful to a low-carb dieter, who needs plenty of protein to keep the body's processes moving along as they should. Mediterranean food also includes plenty of olives, tomatoes, and vegetables, which provide all sorts of vitamins and calcium. Nuts and fruits are also a staple of this type of food, and once again, these are low-carb options for snacks and breakfast.

The only change that is necessary to make from a traditional Mediterranean style diet to a low-carb version of the same is to cut out pasta and bread. Most Mediterranean recipes do include pasta and bread; however, it is simple enough to substitute these items for lower-carb options that can serve the same purpose. For example, instead of a sandwich on bread, try a lettuce wrap with the same filling the sandwich would have had. Instead of pasta, opt for quinoa, which does still have some carbs, but far fewer than the pasta would have. Balance it with a protein for optimal weight loss.

When following a low-carb Mediterranean style diet, it is necessary to keep in mind a few ground rules. To begin with, it is important to remember to eat every two hours on this diet. This helps to balance your blood sugar, and will keep you from crashing at down times throughout the day. However, you should always choose healthy snacks for eating in between meals; have hummus with fresh vegetables or simply a piece of fruit or handful of nuts to keep you going. This way, you will have plenty of extra energy while still not resorting to eating snacks that are too high in carbohydrates. You will also gain lots of extra vitamins by consuming hummus (from the garbanzo beans from which it is made) and fresh veggies, and calcium and other vitamins from the fruit and nuts.

When you do eat carbohydrates, and you should have a very small amount every day, be sure to balance them with plenty of protein. Never have carbohydrates alone, as your body will be less capable of processing them quickly, and this will slow down your metabolism significantly. As mentioned above, it is important to have proteins to keep your body from becoming too tired. If it moves straight from trying to process the few carbs you have ingested to burning fat stores as an energy source, you will feel tired and weak. The protein is necessary as a sort of "middle man" to ensure that you have the energy you need to keep going strong. However, be sure you are eating more than simply proteins, as a protein-only diet is going to cause you problems with digestion and constipation, as well as potentially cause inflammatory bowel disorders. Fiber is necessary to keep your bowels moving as they should and to keep your body flushed out throughout the day.

With any meal or snack, regardless of carbs, always drink lots of water to keep your body flushing everything out regularly in other ways, and to keep yourself well hydrated. Reducing your carbohydrate intake will inevitably cause you to feel more thirsty than you normally would. This is not a bad thing! Everyone can benefit from drinking more water, regardless of whether or not they are dieting or trying to eat low-carb. It is so important to drink plenty of water every day. This can help get rid of excess fat, as well as help you feel better if you are suffering from a cold or allergies.

Avoid caffeinated drinks, carbonated drinks, and alcohol as much as possible, however. Caffeine-free herbal teas are fine to drink, as long as you do not add sugar to them. Otherwise, water is the best choice for drinking.

If you follow these rules, and keep in mind the lists of what to eat and what to avoid in the following chapter, you will be well on your way to significant weight loss through an enjoyable and delicious diet plan that has proven effective for many people already. The recipes in the final few chapters of this book will give you plenty of delicious options to get you started on a road to painless dieting and quick and easy weight loss.

For more information about the paleo style diet, what it includes, what it limits, and how it can help you to lose weight successfully, please see the first two chapters of the book titled

CHAPTER 2 - WHAT TO EAT AND WHAT TO AVOID

When making the switch from your old eating habits to a low-carb, Mediterranean style diet, it is important to focus on proper consumption of food categories. Of course, it goes without saying that you should avoid foods that are high in carbohydrates. But unless a food has a nutrition label from which you can check the carbs, it is difficult to tell what you should and should not eat. The following lists will provide for you some basic information to help you get started on your new diet.

What To Eat

- Fatty fish (salmon, trout, tuna, herring, etc.)
- Walnuts
- Pecans
- Green leafy vegetables
- Olive oil

- Lots of vegetables and fruits every day
- Chicken
- Beef
- Peas
- Beans
- Lentils
- Whole grains
- Eggs

What To Avoid

- Canola oil
- Canned fruits and vegetables
- Overcooked vegetables
- Deli meat
- Refined grains (white bread, white pasta, white rice, etc.)
- Refined sugar
- Margarine
- Pre-packaged commercial foods

Chapter 3 - Sides and Dressings

Vinaigrette

The perfect dressing or flavor addition to any Mediterranean dish. Make this at the beginning of the week to last you up to five days. Making your own vinaigrette takes the guesswork out of purchasing store-bought dressing.

2 tbsp minced garlic

2 tbsp lemon juice

2/3 cup olive oil

4 tbsp fresh parsley

Dash of salt

1 tsp yellow prepared mustard

1 tsp dried paprika

4 tbsp red wine vinegar

1. Chop fresh parsley.
2. In a small bowl, combine all ingredients.
3. Whisk together thoroughly.

4. Let sit for one hour to reach room temperature and blend together flavors.
5. Refrigerate for up to 5 days.
6. Shake well before using.

Kale Side Dish

A tasty and incredibly healthy side dish to pair with any of the dinners in this book. Kale is high in protein and vitamins, and it can give you a boost of energy at any time of the day.

12 cups kale

2 tbsp lemon juice

1 tbsp olive oil

1 tbsp minced garlic

1 tsp soy sauce

Salt and pepper to taste

1. Chop kale.
2. Put a steamer basket in a large saucepan.

3. Fill pan with water to the bottom of the steamer.
4. Cover and bring to a boil.
5. Fill steamer with chopped kale and cover again.
6. Steam for 10 minutes.
7. While steaming, whisk lemon juice, olive oil, garlic, soy sauce, salt and pepper together in a separate bowl.
8. After kale has steamed, toss with dressing and coat thoroughly.

LOW-CARB TZATZIKI SAUCE

Tzatziki is a stale of a Mediterranean diet, and can be a delicious topping for all sorts of vegetables or fish. Make it ahead of time and keep in the refrigerator to use as a topping as you prefer. This recipe only has 5 grams of carbohydrates, so it won't hurt your low-carb diet.

32oz plain low-fat yogurt

1 small cucumber

1 tbsp minced garlic

2 tbsp lemon juice

2 tbsp olive oil

2 tsp lemon zest

3 tbsp dried dill seasoning

Salt and pepper to taste

1. Grate cucumber with peel on.
2. Combine yogurt, cucumber, garlic, lemon juice, and olive oil in a small bowl.
3. Add lemon zest, dill, salt, and pepper.
4. Whisk together all ingredients until dip is smooth.
5. Cover and refrigerate at least 8 hours for flavors to meld.

Homemade Hummus

Tasty with freshly-diced vegetables and low in carbohydrates, hummus can be a great snack or side dish at any time of the day.

2 tbsp minced garlic

16oz can garbanzo beans

4 tbsp lemon juice

2 tbsp tahini

Salt and pepper to taste

2 tbsp olive oil

1. In a blender or food processor, combine minced garlic, garbanzo beans (with liquid—do not drain), lemon juice, tahini, salt, and pepper.
2. Blend or process until completely smooth and creamy.
3. Refrigerate for 2 hours.
4. Top with olive oil before serving.

Chapter 4 - Salads and Lighter Fare

Waldorf-Inspired Salad

A light salad with a summery feel that is sure to make your taste buds happy.

2 apples of any variety

3 celery stalks

1 cup chopped walnuts

Salt and pepper to taste

2 tbsp walnut oil

1 tbsp cider vinegar

Dash of cinnamon

Dash of nutmeg

1. Dice apples and celery.
2. Combine oil, vinegar, cinnamon and nutmeg in a small lidded container and shake until well mixed.
3. Place diced apples, celery, and chopped walnuts in a bowl.
4. Cover with dressing and toss to cover thoroughly and evenly.
5. Chill for an hour before serving.

TURKEY TOMATO BOWL

Full of protein and vitamins, this recipe is easy to make ahead of time and take with you on the go.

6oz pre-cooked unseasoned diced turkey

2 small tomatoes

2 tbsp balsamic vinaigrette

Black pepper to taste

1oz roasted macadamia nuts

1. Dice tomatoes.
2. Place turkey and tomato in a microwave-safe bowl.
3. Top with vinaigrette.
4. Microwave for 80 seconds.
5. Add black pepper as desired.
6. Sprinkle with macadamia nuts and serve.

Chicken Topped Salad

This recipe will taste like it took hours to make, when in reality, it's very quick and easy.

8oz raw chicken breast tenderloin

1/4 cup canned mandarin orange wedges in light syrup

Dash of lemon pepper seasoning

4oz romaine lettuce

1oz baby spinach

1 small cucumber

1 small Haas avocado

1 small tomato

1oz walnuts

6 tbsp olive oil

2 tbsp balsamic vinegar

Dash dried rosemary

Salt and pepper to taste

1. Peel and dice cucumber, avocado, and tomato.
2. Cook chicken breast in a skillet over medium heat for 10 minutes.

3. While chicken is cooking, combine olive oil, vinegar, salt, pepper, and rosemary in a lidded jar and shake to combine.
4. Tear lettuce and spinach into smaller pieces and arrange on a plate.
5. Add cucumber, avocado, tomato, cooked chicken, walnuts, and orange wedges to the lettuce and spinach.
6. Top with vinaigrette mixture.

BLT Wraps

A low-carb take on an old favorite!

1 Haas avocado

6 strips thick-sliced bacon

4oz romaine lettuce

1 medium tomato

1oz pecans

1. Peel and slice avocado.
2. Cook bacon over medium heat to preferred doneness.
3. Lay out some of the romaine lettuce leaves.

4. Top lettuce with bacon, tomato, and avocado.

5. Repeat for remaining lettuce.

6. Fold and serve with a side of pecans.

CHICKEN FAJITA LETTUCE WRAPS

Like the BLT wraps, this wrap makes use of romaine lettuce instead of bread or tortillas, which keeps the carbs very low.

1 pound boneless skinless chicken breast

1 small onion

1 green bell pepper

1 red bell pepper

2 tbsp olive oil

1 medium tomato

Salt and pepper to taste

1 tsp chili powder

1 tsp dried parsley flakes

Dash dried oregano

Dash dried cumin

Dash dried paprika

1/3 cup water

16oz romaine lettuce

4oz walnuts

4 small pears

1. Dice onion, red and green bell peppers, and tomato.
2. Cut chicken breast into strips.
3. Cook onions and peppers in 1 tbsp olive oil in a skillet over medium-high heat for 10 minutes.
4. Remove vegetables and set aside.
5. Cook chicken in 1 tbsp olive oil in skillet over medium-high heat for 5 to 7 minutes.
6. Add water and spices to skillet.
7. Bring to a boil, then turn heat to low and simmer for 4 minutes.
8. Place spoonfuls of mixture atop leaves of romaine lettuce.
9. Fold and enjoy with a side of walnuts and pear.

Light Salad

This salad is easy on the stomach. The ingredients used to prepare it make it a perfect option for detox or for days when you might be dealing with digestive inflammation.

1 small cucumber

2 tbsp lemon juice

2 tbsp olive oil

Black pepper to taste

6 cups romaine lettuce

14oz can artichoke hearts

2 large celery stalks

1 small red onion

1/2 cup feta cheese

1. Slice cucumber and celery stalks.
2. Dice onion.
3. Drain and quarter artichoke hearts.
4. Place cucumber and lemon juice in blender or food processor and mix well.
5. Pour olive oil and pulse until combined with cucumber and lemon juice.

6. Season with black pepper.
7. Place romaine, artichoke hearts, celery, red onion, and feta cheese in a bowl.
8. Toss with blended dressing to coat thoroughly.

STUFFED TOMATOES

On the verge between light and hearty. The tomatoes give you plenty of vitamins, while the cheese and olives add calcium.

2 large tomatoes

1/2 cup pre-packaged garlic croutons

1/4 cup goat cheese

1/4 cup sliced kalamata olives

2 tbsp vinaigrette

2 tbsp fresh thyme

1. Chop fresh thyme.
2. Cut tomatoes in half and remove seeds and pulp.
3. Save pulp in a separate bowl.

4. Add croutons, goat cheese, olives, vinaigrette, and thyme to pulp and combine thoroughly.
5. Spoon mixture into hollowed tomatoes.
6. Place tomatoes on a broiler pan.
7. Broil for 5 minutes.

Garbanzo Bean Salad

Very light and extra-tasty. This salad is so simple and delicious, you will want it every day of the week.

9oz package precooked unseasoned diced chicken breast

15oz can chickpeas

1 small cucumber

4 green onions

1/4 cup fresh basil

1/2 cup plain fat-free yogurt

2 tbsp minced garlic

Pinch of salt

2 cups baby spinach

1/3 cup feta cheese

4 lemon wedges

1. Drain chickpeas.
2. Peel and dice cucumber and dice green onions.
3. Chop basil.
4. Gently combine chicken breast, chickpeas, cucumber, green onions, basil, yogurt, garlic, and salt.
5. Add spinach and feta to mixture.
6. Serve garnished with lemon wedges to squeeze over salad.

Tuna Salad

A classic! This recipe is great for kids and adults both.

12oz canned tuna

1/4 cup low-fat mayonnaise

1/4 cup chopped black olives

1/4 cup roasted red peppers

2 green onions

1 tbsp capers

Romaine lettuce

1. Drain and flake canned tuna.
2. Chop roasted red peppers and green onions.
3. Drain capers.
4. Combine ingredients except lettuce in a bowl and mix thoroughly.
5. Serve tuna salad over lettuce leaves or as a lettuce wrap.

QUINOA SALAD

Enjoy plenty of Mediterranean flavors in this unique lunchtime treat.

2 cups water

2 cubes chicken bouillon

2 tbsp minced garlic

1 cup uncooked quinoa

1 package unseasoned pre-cooked diced chicken breast

1 large red onion

1 green bell pepper

1/2 cup chopped kalamata olives

1/2 cup feta cheese

1/4 cup fresh parsley

1/4 cup green onions

Dash of salt

2/3 cup lemon juice

1 tbsp balsamic vinegar

1/4 cup olive oil

1. Dice red onion, bell pepper, parsley, and green onions.
2. Boil water, bouillon cubes, and garlic over medium-high heat in a pot.
3. Add in quinoa.
4. Reduce heat to low and simmer for 20 minutes.
5. Remove from heat.
6. Mix chicken, onion, bell pepper, olives, feta cheese, parsley, green onion, and salt into quinoa.
7. Drizzle with lemon juice, balsamic vinegar, and olive oil.
8. Mix thoroughly.
9. Chill for 1 hour before serving.

Simple Caprese Salad

So simple, so quick, and such a tasty lunch!

4 large tomatoes

1 pound fresh mozzarella

1/3 cup fresh basil

3 tbsp olive oil

Salt and pepper to taste

1. Slice tomatoes and mozzarella cheese.
2. Chop basil.
3. Arrange tomato slices, mozzarella slices, and basil leaves on a plate.
4. Drizzle with olive oil.
5. Sprinkle with salt and pepper.

Halibut Salad

12oz skinned halibut filets

Salt and pepper to taste

3 tbsp olive oil

1 tbsp minced garlic

1/4 cup low-fat mayonnaise

1/4 cup sun-dried tomatoes

1/4 cup fresh basil

2 tbsp fresh parsley

1 tbsp capers

1 large lemon

4 cups arugula

1. Preheat oven to 450 degrees Fahrenheit.

2. Chop sun-dried tomatoes, fresh basil, and fresh parsley.

3. Drain and mash capers; zest lemon.

4. Season halibut with salt and pepper to taste.

5. Rub fish with olive oil.

6. Place in a baking dish and bake for 15 minutes.

7. Let fish cool.

8. In a separate bowl, mix mayonnaise, tomatoes, basil, parsley, capers, and zest from lemon. Combine well.

9. Flake halibut into bowl.

10. Mix fish into mayonnaise mixture thoroughly.

11. Serve on top of arugula.

Chapter 5 - Heartier Meals

Mediterranean Chicken

This recipe is a classic dinnertime favorite sure to please the whole family.

2 tsp olive oil

2 tbsp white wine

6 chicken breast halves

3 tbsp minced garlic

1 small onion

3 small tomatoes

2 tsp fresh thyme

1 tbsp fresh basil

1/2 cup sliced kalamata olives

1/4 cup fresh parsley

Salt and pepper to taste

1. Dice onion and tomatoes.
2. Chop fresh thyme, fresh basil, and fresh parsley.
3. Heat olive oil and 2 tbsp white wine in skillet over medium heat.

4. Add chicken to oil and wine in skillet.
5. Saute for 5 minutes; turn over and sauté other side for 5 minutes.
6. Remove chicken from skillet.
7. In pan drippings, saute garlic for 1 minute.
8. Add onion and tomatoes and bring to a boil.
9. Reduce heat to low.
10. Add 1/2 cup white wine and simmer on low for 10 minutes.
11. Add thyme and basil; simmer for 5 more minutes on low.
12. Return chicken to skillet and cover.
13. Simmer until chicken is cooked through.
14. Add olives and parsley and cook for 1 more minute.
15. Season with salt and pepper as desired.

STEAK AND OLIVES

This recipe is light on the ingredients but hearty and filling.

5oz thin round steak

1 Haas avocado

14 pitted black olives

1 medium tomato

Salt and pepper to taste

1. Slice avocado and tomato.
2. Sprinkle salt and pepper on steak as desired.
3. Cook steak over medium heat in a skillet for 1 to 2 minutes per side.
4. Arrange steak on a plate with sliced avocado, black olives, and sliced tomato.
5. Serve.

BASIC BREAKFAST

A delicious breakfast option that never gets old!

3 eggs

3 thick-sliced bacon strips

Salt and pepper to taste

1/2 cup raw honeydew melon

1. Fry bacon over medium heat to desired doneness.
2. Fry eggs over medium heat to desired doneness.
3. For sunny side up eggs, do not flip; for all others, flip halfway through cooking with a rubber spatula.
4. Slice honeydew melon into cubes.
5. Serve.

SHISH-KABOB SKEWERS

It doesn't get much more Mediterranean than a shish-kabob. Keep it low carb with this favorite.

1/2 cup tomato juice

2 tbsp vodka

Dash Worcestershire sauce

2 stalks celery

Salt and pepper to taste

Grape tomatoes

Artichoke hearts

Kalamata olives

Dash tabasco sauce

1/4 teaspoon horseradish

2 tbsp olive oil

1. Dice celery.
2. Combine tomato juice, vodka, Worcestershire, tabasco, horseradish, oil, celery, salt and pepper with a whisk in a small bowl.
3. Refrigerate mixture until ready to serve.
4. Skewer a grape tomato, artichoke heart, and black olive on each skewer.
5. Optional: include small mozzarella balls on skewers as well.
6. Serve with vinaigrette.

CHICKPEA PATTIES

For a healthy, low-carb burger night with a tangy flair!

15oz can chickpeas

1/2 cup fresh parsley

1 tbsp minced garlic

1/4 tsp ground cumin

Salt and pepper to taste

1 egg

4 tbsp all-purpose flour

2 tbsp olive oil

1/2 cup low-fat Greek yogurt

3 tbsp lemon juice

8 cups romaine lettuce

1 small red onion

1 cup grape tomatoes

1. Drain and rinse chickpeas
2. Whisk egg.
3. Dice onion.
4. Combine chickpeas, parsley, garlic, and cumin in a food processor or blender and chop.
5. Pour mixture into a bowl.
6. Add whisked egg and 2 tbsp flour and mix well.
7. Form into 8 patties.

8. Roll patties in remaining flour.
9. Cook patties in olive oil over medium-high heat for 3 minutes per side.
10. Combine yogurt, lemon juice, and salt and pepper in a small bowl with a whisk.
11. Arrange 4 servings of lettuce, tomatoes, onion, and chickpea patties on plates.
12. Drizzle with dressing.

Simple and Delicious Salmon

This fishy fare is full of protein and Omega-3s. It's an excellent dinner choice for a Friday night.

4 (6oz) salmon filets

2 cups cherry tomatoes

1 small zucchini

2 tbsp capers

1 tbsp olive oil

1 small can sliced black olives

Salt and pepper to taste

1. Halve cherry tomatoes.
2. Peel and thinly slice zucchini.
3. Drain and rinse capers and black olives.
4. Preheat oven to 425 degrees Fahrenheit.
5. Sprinkle salt and pepper on fish as desired.
6. Place in a baking dish.
7. Mix tomatoes, zucchini, capers, olive oil, and black olives in a small bowl.
8. Spoon tomato mixture over fish in baking dish.
9. Bake for 20 minutes in preheated oven.

STUFFED MUSHROOMS

Make a traditional appetizer a fully balanced meal with this low-carb offering.

4 large portobello mushrooms

1/2 a small onion

1 celery stalk

1/2 a carrot

1/2 a green bell pepper

1/2 a red bell pepper

Dash dried Italian seasoning mix

2 tbsp minced garlic

3 cups pre-packaged garlic croutons

1/2 cup vegetable broth

1/2 cup feta cheese

3 tbsp balsamic vinaigrette

4 tsp grated fresh Parmesan cheese

Dash black pepper

4 cups romaine lettuce

1. Finely dice onion, celery, carrot, and green and red bell peppers.
2. Preheat oven to 350 degrees Fahrenehti.
3. Remove stems from mushrooms and finely dice stems.
4. Combine stems, onion, celery, carrot, green bell pepper, red bell pepper, Italian seasoning, and minced garlic in a small bowl.
5. Transfer mixture to a skillet and cook for 10 minutes over medium heat.

6. Remove to a large bowl and add croutons; combine thoroughly.
7. Add broth slowly to mixture and toss to coat thoroughly.
8. Add feta cheese and toss again.
9. Remove and discard gills from mushroom caps.
10. Place mushroom caps on a baking sheet and brush evenly with vinaigrette.
11. Sprinkle Parmesan and pepper over mushrooms.
12. Top each mushroom with bread mixture.
13. Bake mushrooms in preheated oven for 25 minutes.
14. Place romaine lettuce on plates and top with mushrooms.

ROASTED RED PEPPER

Perfect for parties and get-togethers, this recipe is healthy and incredibly filling.

6 large red bell peppers

1 tbsp olive oil

4 tbsp minced garlic

6oz fresh spinach

1 tbsp lemon juice

Dash of salt

3/4 cup uncooked couscous

1/2 cup feta cheese

1. Roast bell peppers on a rack under the oven's broiler for 15 minutes. Turn every 5 minutes.
2. Transfer to a bowl and cool.
3. After cooling, peel peppers and cut off the tops.
4. Rinse out seeds from peppers and set aside.
5. Sauté garlic for 1 minute in olive oil over medium-high heat.
6. Add spinach and turn down heat to medium.
7. Cook for 2 minutes or until spinach is wilted.
8. Remove from heat.

9. Add lemon juice and salt and transfer to a small bowl.
10. Preheat oven to 350 degrees Fahrenheit.
11. Cook couscous on the stovetop or microwave according to package directions.
12. Add cooked couscous and feta cheese to spinach mixture and mix thoroughly.
13. Stuff peppers with couscous stuffing and place on a baking sheet lined with tinfoil.
14. Bake on center rack for 8 minutes.
15. Serve warm.

ROSEMARY CHICKEN

Have this low-carb dish for a fancy dinner or serve it as a weekly meal. Either way, it is simple and flavorful.

1 small onion

1 medium red bell pepper

4 tbsp minced garlic

2 tsp dried rosemary

1/2 tsp dried oregano

8oz Italian turkey sausage

32oz chicken breasts

Salt and pepper to taste

1/4 cup dry vermouth

1-1/2 tbsp cornstarch

2 tbsp cold water

1/4 cup fresh parsley

1. Dice onion and red bell pepper.
2. Chop parsley.
3. Remove casings from turkey sausage.
4. In a slow cooker, place onion, bell pepper, garlic, rosemary, and oregano.
5. Crumble sausage (casings removed) over spices in slow cooker.
6. Rinse chicken, dry, and place over sausage crumbles in slow cooker.
7. Season with salt and pepper as desired.
8. Add vermouth.

9. Cook on low for 7 hours, then remove chicken from slow cooker.

10. In a small bowl, combine cornstarch and cold water.

11. Stir mixture into liquid and sausage remaining in slow cooker.

12. Increase temperature to high setting and cook for 10 minutes, stirring twice.

13. Season sauce with salt and pepper as desired.

14. Pour sauce over chicken.

15. Sprinkle with parsley.

Chapter 6 - Weekly Meal Plan and Daily Shopping Lists

- For a successful Low-Carb Mediterranean style kitchen, there are a few items which you will want to keep in stock in your pantry or refrigerator at all times. You will use these items every day, or at least almost every day, so be sure to purchase them weekly or keep your supplies up:
- Olive oil
- Lemon juice
- Romaine lettuce
- Minced garlic
- Fresh thyme
- Fresh basil
- Fresh parsley
- Dried cinnamon
- Dried nutmeg
- Dried parsley

- Dried oregano
- Dried cumin
- Dried paprika
- Dried rosemary
- Feta cheese

Monday

Breakfast - Bacon and Melon

Lunch - Waldorf-Inspired Salad

Dinner - Mediterranean Chicken

Shopping List

Thick-sliced bacon

Cantaloupe or honeydew melon

2 medium apples, any variety

Celery

Raw walnuts

Walnut oil

Cider vinegar

White wine

6 boneless skinless chicken breasts

Small onion

2 medium tomatoes

Kalamata olives

Tuesday

Breakfast - 1/2 Large Grapefruit

Lunch - Chicken Fajita Lettuce Wraps

Dinner - Steak and Olives

Shopping List

Large grapefruit

1 pound boneless chicken breast

Medium onion

One green and one red bell pepper

2 large tomatoes

Chili powder

Raw walnuts

4 small pears

5oz thin round steak

1 Haas avocado

Pitted canned black olives

Wednesday

Breakfast - Bacon and Melon

Lunch - Light Salad

Dinner - Shish-kabob Skewers

Shopping List

- Thick-sliced bacon
- Cantaloupe or honeydew melon
- Large cucumber
- 14oz canned artichoke hearts
- Celery
- Small red onion
- Tomato juice
- Vodka
- Worcestershire sauce
- Celery
- Grape tomatoes
- 14oz canned artichoke hearts
- Pitted canned kalamata olives
- Tabasco sauce
- Horseradish

Thursday

- Breakfast - 1/2 Large Grapefruit
- Lunch - Turkey Tomato Bowl
- Dinner - Chickpea Patties

Shopping List

Large grapefruit

Pre-cooked unseasoned diced turkey

1 medium tomato

Low-fat vinaigrette (or pre-make vinaigrette recipe included in this book)

Roasted macadamia nuts

16oz canned chickpeas

Eggs

All-purpose flour

Small container plain Greek yogurt

Grape tomatoes

Small red onion

Friday

Breakfast - Bacon and Melon

Lunch - Chicken Topped Salad

Dinner - Simple and Delicious Salmon

Shopping List

Thick-sliced bacon

Cantaloupe or honeydew melon

8oz raw chicken breast tenderloin

Canned mandarin orange wedges in light syrup

Lemon pepper seasoning

Baby spinach

1 small cucumber

Haas avocado

Small tomato

Raw walnuts

Vinegar

24oz salmon filets

Grape tomatoes

1 large zucchini

Small can capers

Canned sliced black olives

Saturday

Breakfast - Basic Breakfast

Lunch - Garbanzo Bean Salad

Dinner - Stuffed Mushrooms

Shopping List

Eggs

Thick-sliced bacon

Honeydew melon

Package pre-cooked unseasoned diced chicken breast

15oz canned chickpeas

1 small cucumber

Bundle green onions

Small container of plain fat-free yogurt

Package of baby spinach

1 lemon

4 large portobello mushroom caps

Small onion

Celery

1 carrot

1 red and 1 green bell pepper

Italian seasoning

Packaged croutons

Vegetable broth

Low-fat vinaigrette (or pre-make vinaigrette recipe included in this book)

Grated Parmesan cheese

Sunday

Breakfast - BLT Wraps

Lunch - Stuffed Tomatoes

Dinner - Rosemary Chicken

Shopping List

Medium Haas avocado

Thick-sliced bacon

Raw pecans

3 large tomatoes

Packaged garlic croutons

Goat cheese

Sliced kalamata olives

Low-fat vinaigrette (or pre-make vinaigrette recipe included in this book)

Small onion

1 red bell pepper

8oz Italian turkey sausage

32oz skinless boneless chicken breast

Cornstarch

Conclusion

Thank you again for downloading this book!

I hope this book was able to help you to understand the basics of a low-carb Mediterranean style diet, and get inspired by the many delicious recipes provided here.

The next step is to go shopping and start cooking!

About The Author

Conrad Spencer is born with the vision to promote the art of *Low Carb* among the masses. The author has written several research papers on the topic. He has served as an instructor promoting various cultural arts in University of San Francisco. He is currently living with his spouse in Texas.

www.ingramcontent.com/pod-product-compliance
Lightning Source LLC
LaVergne TN
LVHW020427080526
838202LV00055B/5059